KYNDRA JOHNSON

Gut Health Hacks For Beginners

Free Yourself From The Effects Of Poor Gut Health With Tips From Someone Who's Been There Before

First edition

This book was professionally typeset on Reedsy.
Find out more at reedsy.com

Contents

1

Introduction

If you're reading this I'm guessing that either yourself or someone you love is battling through the trenches of what it is to have poor gut health. The kind of gut that is wreaking havoc on your body and manifesting itself in more than a few ways. Affecting your quality of life, and has you wondering if you'll ever experience feeling "normal" ever again.

I know this is how you're probably feeling because I've been there too. Oh have I been there. My name is Kyndra Johnson and I have experienced and learned from what it means to have a "leaky Gut". I consider that time one of the darkest and most difficult in my life because of the way my unhealthy gut not just troubled me physically but mentally as well.

Now, I wouldn't be writing this book if I was still in the depths of confusion and discomfort, and hadn't found methods that helped me overcome this major obstacle in my life. I'm here because I HAVE. My purpose in writing this is to offer a comprehensive guide of first steps and achievable advice that I wish would have been summed up for me at the beginning of my healing journey. In order for you to understand the weight this carries with me, and why I have such a passion for educating others on the matter. Let me tell you how I got here.

2

My story

It was May of 2021 when I was vacationing in Cabo with my family that it all began. I had eaten a large dinner of the most tender beef I've had in my entire life. Later that night as I slept I was awoken by intense nausea. I already don't handle nausea well. It brings me a lot of anxiety which no doubt makes it worse. But this nausea was different from any other bout I've had. It was debilitating. I thought for sure if I was able to throw up I would feel better, but I never actually could. I don't even know if you could call it nausea at this point. It had to be something different entirely,but for the sake of explanation that's the closest description to it. It lasted the vast majority of the night and by morning I was feeling much better. I chalked it up to being something bad that I ate from dinner and moved on. Not so.

We were only half way through our all inclusive trip at this point and there was more food to be eaten. The next morning I ate breakfast and a few hours later I found myself doubled over with the same intense sickness from the night before. For the rest of the trip every time I ate anything I was sick a few hours later. In hindsight I can see that these episodes started at the time my body would have started digesting the food. Now I know what you might be thinking. You were pregnant!

This was a thought I had as well as it came on so suddenly and felt like the only explanation. After getting home from my trip the episodes continued. I waited for the time I was able to take a pregnancy test to see if this was the reason behind my incredible and out of nowhere discomfort and poor health. If you could guess, the test was negative. Now here I am a few weeks later now in a state of malnutrition from lack of eating and the only explanation I had lined up was proven not to be the reason.

Now if you can imagine this went on for the next year. I ended up in the ER twice for intense chest pain that they chalked up to be heartburn after taking EKGs. I was already a small individual with a starting weight of 135. By this time I had gotten to a staggering 112 pounds. I would go days without eating just to have those days broken up by my small bowls of rice. I later started cooking the rice in chicken broth and added salt to achieve the flavor that I so desperately longed for. In that year I saw multiple doctors, and spent thousands of dollars on testing just to be told there was nothing physically wrong with me. I even had one doctor who had the audacity to tell me it was anxiety and recommend medication. Here we have a prime example of a doctor who pushed medications to cover up symptoms instead of investigating a root cause. I left feeling completely and utterly alone. No one could help me. I was out of money, and I was out of hope.

I remember specifically a time that whole year later on a summer evening out on my parents boat. It was sunset and we decided to turn up the music and just cruise for a while. I remember vividly, my husband holding me in his arms with my eyes fixed on my 2 small beautiful children and thinking to myself. This is it. I'm going to die and no one is going to know why. It was a sobering moment to say the least. I looked up at my husband with tear filled eyes and told him how much I loved him.

A few months later we found ourselves visiting some friends we hadn't seen in a while. After telling my friend of my struggles she asked me if I had ever heard of a hair DNA analysis scan. Essentially they take a strand of your hair and they scan it to some device that reads your hair and sends results over to Germany for inspection. Within a few minutes you have a 30 page report on your overall health. My mind was blown. I thought, what's 250 more dollars? If it meant I might find some answers.

I scheduled something and was getting my own scan done within a week. A birds eye view of this test showed your body's levels of interference or the levels of 50 HZ main currents such as the effects of computer monitors, microwave ovens, mobile telephones, wifi, ect. It showed the different amounts and types of amino acids, fatty acids, minerals, environmental challenges, antioxidants, and food sensitivities. For the first time in my life I had seen that there was so much more to a wholesome and healthy body than just food, and exercise. Calories and macro nutrients.

Of the major points in my results it showed that the biggest imbalances were in my detoxification system, gut and intestinal, as well as emotion, sugar and metabolism. After going through the results with my tech she had introduced to me something I had never heard of in my life. " Have you ever heard of the term Leaky Gut." she asked me. Of course my answer was no and she began to educate me on what it was and of the possibility that it could be the root cause of all of my symptoms. A familiar spark was lit inside of me. A spark that had slowly faded and ran out over the year of complete darkness. Everything in my heart and mind told me this was it. Learning about and healing my gut at its core was going to be what lifted me from this curse.

If you haven't guessed by now. We were right. From here the research began. The *work* began. And today in 2024 I stand before you a whole, healthy, and happy human being with the chershiment of my new knowledge that I have that healed me and has been able to get others on the track to their healing as well. If you want this to be your story. I plead with you to not only finish this book but also put into action the advice and tips that I offer as they were the basic steps I took in my own life to not just heal my gut but my body as a whole.

3

What Is Leaky Gut and How Can it Affect You

Before we dive into all the nitty gritty of what we can do to heal our guts and our bodies one must first understand what the condition means. So that the advice and tips I offer hold more weight. So that they make sense to you.

Leaky gut is often referred to as intestinal permeability. In fact doctors will take you more seriously if you refer to it as this. And it is essentially how it sounds. Perforations on the intestines large enough to allow toxins and undigested food in the intestines to escape and travel to your bloodstream creating a chemical reaction or an inflammatory response. This explained why I got sick everytime I ate. Even if was a mere carrot stick,

Symptoms can manifest as nausea with or without vomiting, bloating, abdominal discomfort, decreased immunity, food sensitivities, indigestion, burning feeling in gut, diarrhea, chronic fatigue, skin irritations such as acne, psoriasis, and eczema, joint pain, brain fog, depression, anxiety and other mood disorders. If you can relate to any of these problems chances are something in your gut needs to be addressed.

4

What Causes Leaky Gut?

So What caused those perforations to happen in the first place? There are a few factors but the most common is chronic inflammation. Chronic inflammation is a natural and necessary function of the body's immune response to harmful stimuli, infection, or injury. Chronic means that it has been present over an extended period of time, and the immune system may start attacking healthy tissues. If the intestinal barrier has eroded it most likely didn't happen overnight. The most common chronic inflammatory conditions come from or include IBD, IBS, celiac, HIV, AIDS, Chemotherapy, overuse of alcohol and NSAIDS such as tylenol and ibuprofen and food allergies as which cause an immune response which in turn activates the body's response to increase inflammation.

Not only are conditions such as these potential perpetrators but the American lifestyle is no doubt a contributing factor that is constantly triggering our bodies' immune and inflammatory responses. With the typical American diet being a low fiber, high in polyunsaturated fats, and artificial foods that can only be conjured up in a lab. Along with the overuse of alcohol, medications, and high stress lifestyles. No wonder our bodies are deteriorating from the inside out. We're not giving them a chance without even realizing it because this has become the "normal" way of life. Subsequently if you do different you're labeled as either a loony or a hippie.

5

First Things To Stop Doing

Now let's get down to the nitty gritty shall we? You've identified these symptoms in yourself and have most likely related to me and my story in some way. You bought this book because you have the desire and have seen the need to clean up, and restore your gut health to get you on track to feeling better, lighter, more energized and in a lot of cases pain free.

Let's talk about the first things you need to stop doing. And I mean cold turkey. I'm not going to beat around the bush here. This is going to take some work, some discipline, some patience, and a whole lot of dedication. After all, you are healing potentially decades of damage. If you were anything like me I would have done whatever it took if it meant I could start to eat without the fear of a major episode. Or have the energy to play with my kids and enjoy life the way I had before or even better.

First things first. We must decrease the inflammation in our bodies. A huge factor to this is our diet. We gotta stop with the polyunsaturated oils or PUFAS for short. You may have heard of these. All the influencers these days refer to these fireballs as "seed oils". We're talking vegetable oil, canola oil, rapeseed oil, sunflower oil, safflower oil, flax seed oil, and rapeseed oils. However there are certain oils that will be beneficial to the building back up for our gut health which we will get into a bit later. I guarantee you. If you went and picked out any packaged product in your pantry 90% or more of them are guaranteed to have some sort of PUFA in them. The reason? Because they're cheap. Big business likes cheap. Don't let them fool you. They truly care more about their buck than your health. The sad part is, so many products will mis label and advertise something as being a "healthy option". When in reality they have a mile long list of ingredients conjured in a lab at the cheapest price. They can say whatever they want about their product there is no one managing or regulating for that. The food industry is especially sneaky in America. Did you know a large percentage of the food we consume in America is banned in most other countries? Skittles, Twinkies, Pillsbury Biscuits, Mountain Dew, Frosted flakes, Fruit Loops to name a few. Keeping in mind that some of the worst of them are advertised towards children. It honestly makes me sick. Other than PUFAS you're also going to want to cut out all preservatives, artificial sweeteners, food dyes, and high fructose corn syrups.

There are 3 main rules I follow when I go shopping. That is, if I don't recognize an ingredient it's a no. I Would also ask myself if I could make this product with ingredients in my kitchen. At the beginning of my journey I knew not a lick of what was on the back of labels or what the heck any of it meant.

For my third rule my general consensus was that if it had more than 10 ingredients it was a no for me. Now as you progress in your journey and continue to do your own research and practice, the label reading will start to come naturally. In fact it's become a really fun hobby for myself and even my husband. We find ourselves looking to the back of labels just for the fun of it to see how outrageous some of these ingredient lists are. If you want to know what I'm talking about, take a look at any store shelf syrup that's not 100 percent pure maple syrup and you will see exactly what I mean.

Something else you should stop doing immediately is diary and gluten. Now I'm not saying permanently. But while you're working to bring down the inflammation this could help immensely as these are both very inflammatory foods. If you really feel like this is something you would struggle with. A fantastic alternative to bread and baked goods would be sour dough. Especially since sourdough contains crucial probiotics needed to create that healthy gut microbiome that's needed to rebuild tissue and make your mad tummy a happy tummy. For dairy, I would suggest looking into the benefits of raw milk.

I could write an entire chapter about why store bought milk is inflammatory, and why raw milk is not something to be feared but I'll sum it up by saying this. Those who experience lactose intolerance are having a reaction to lactose. Lactose is not naturally digested by our bodies which is why a lot of people have a hard time digesting it. It's supposed to be accompanied by the enzyme lactase which breaks down that lactose enzyme allowing our bodies to digest it. So where did the lactase go? It was burned out in homogenization. So many of the crucial vitamins, minerals and nutrients that are foundational in the creation of milk are stripped away in that Homogenization and pasteurization process. That's why you see a lot of whole milk advertised with "added Vitamin D" . They are having to replace that vitamin that was lost with yet another artificial form of ingredient. So, raw milk. Look into it if you really feel like dairy is going to be a deal breaker for you.

Something else you should stop doing right away are eating in large portions. Portion control is huge. It's common sense really. Think about it. Your body is struggling to digest as it is and you're shoveling large amounts of food into your digestive system. It's not going to handle it well if it's in a state of repair.

Let's recap. If you were going to stop doing any 5 things to lower the inflammation in your gut and start on your road to recovery it would be this. Throw out the PUFAS, eliminate refined, processed sugars, as well as preservatives and artificial ingredients. Temporarily eliminate or reduce dairy and gluten and start sizing down on your portions. If you just stopped doing these 5 things not only would your gut get started on the road to recovery but so would your overall health.

6

Things You Should Start Doing

Now that we've gone over the first steps of things you should stop doing. Let's go over some simple but substantial things you should start doing. I'll say it again and again. We've got to get this inflammation under control if you want to start seeing results. As mentioned before, inflammation in large part has a lot to do with our diet. So first things first. Get started on that whole food diet. Foods that can be grown or made in your very own home. If you don't know what it is, don't eat it. Next we have got to start reducing stress.

Research estimated that as much as 90 percent of illness and disease is stress related. That's crazy to think about but it makes so much sense and helps you understand what stress can mean on the body.

When you are chronically stressed your body is in a phase of constant fight or flight mode. Meaning your cortisol levels are always at an all time high and don't come down. Your body's protective mechanism is inflammation. Much like how your body produces a fever to fight a detected virus or illness. Therefore high levels of stress definitely contribute to inflammation all throughout the body.

Recommendations for decreasing stress are prayer, meditation, journaling, breathing exercises or anything you feel helps ground you.

I'm a strong believer in taking your life into your own hands. If you don't like your circumstances. Change them. If you have a high stress job or you're stuck doing something you don't love. Change that. No matter your circumstances or the cards you've been dealt. At the end of the day our decisions are our own. Each individual has the power and the god given right to choose and make decisions for oneself. So there you go. If you're in a lifestyle or situation that is causing a chronic amount of stress. Do something about it.

The other kind of less talked about stress is physical stress. Which occurs when our bodies recognize something that is not naturally supposed to be there. We stuff our bodies with these stresses all day everyday without even realizing it. That Teflon you cook on? Leaks forever metals into the food you cook on it. That air freshener or candle you love so much has fragrance in it which is just the short way of listing hundreds or thousands of different kinds of chemicals.

Medications that are filled with fillers and artificial versions of things our bodies should be making on their own but are not in a condition to do so. NSAIDS are a huge one since they are over the counter and can be taken everyday at the first sight or feeling of any discomfort in the body which, by the way, always has a root cause that is being shoved to the side and ignored because of the ability to just cover them up with medications. Which in turn can just add to the stress load of an already stressed body. The end of those medication commercials where it's listing out all the possible side effects is running through my mind right now.

The next thing you can start doing is feeding that gut microbiome by increasing food diversity, taking a good quality pre and probiotic as well as introducing more fermented food that naturally have the awesome pre and probiotics in them. Foods such as sourdough as mentioned before. Yogurt, sauerkraut, kimchi, kefir, apple cider vinegar, miso, kombucha to name a few. We'll get into the gut microbiome a bit more in a future chapter.

Lastly, increase your fiber and stay hydrated. Doing so will keep things moving as smoothly as possible. Detoxification also plays a major role in gut health. And pooping is literally our bodies way of ridding our bodies of toxins. If it doesn't they all just stay and fester causing a whole slew of issues. If you're not having a bowel movement once a day that is definitely a priority. Twice is even better. For simplicity sake the first actions I recommend you start doing right away would be working on reducing inflammation with a whole food diet and reducing stress. You're also going to want to feed that gut microbiome, and increase fiber and hydration. Simple right!?

7

Resources Of Knowledge That Opened My Eyes

There were two main resources that really got my gears moving to the world of taking action on whole body health and wellness. One was the instagram account @justingredients. She is a wealth of knowledge when starting out in your whole food diet, and learning of the importance of finding natural products. Her podcast has remained my top 3 most listened to. I just love learning from her. The second most impactful resource was the podcast called @freelyrooted. It was here that I discovered the discussion of finding the root causes of our issues and then the world of pro metabolic eating which is the approach of eating I used to heal and continue to remain healthy with today.

At its core pro metabolic eating is the process of reducing inflammation and stress in the body by nourishing it with easy to digest, bio available, nutrient dense foods. Simply put, the 5 major elements to this way of life are

1. Eating easily digestible and bio available foods
2. Eating more, not less. More because our bodies need nourishment

17

to perform the way they were designed. One of our bodies' designs is to be able to heal itself from ailments. My suggestion in the beginning was to eat smaller portions more frequently, not just *eating less*.

3. Never skip breakfast
4. Balance your fats
5. Eat seasonally.

May I stress that this is not a diet but a lifestyle. A lifestyle that has allowed me to not just maintain my gut health but feel energized, have better immunity, and maintain an optimal and healthy weight.

8

Foods To Avoid

If you're looking for some more cut and dry type advice and are still feeling like you have no idea where to start. May I suggest a list of types of foods to avoid right here and now. Condensed into an easy refer back to list.

-Processed foods high in additives, preservatives

-PUFAS or "seed oils"

-refined sugar

-gluten (potentially temporarily)

-dairy (potentially temporarily)

-fried foods

-alcohol

-caffeine

-high fructose corn syrup

-spicy foods

-acidic foods

9

Foods To Start Including

We've talked about what foods to avoid now let's talk about what would be a good idea to start including.

-Foods high in glutamine which is an amino acid found in animal and plant proteins including meat, fish, spinach, cabbage, nuts, and beans.

Glutamine has been proven to aid in the healing and maintaining the intestinal lining.

-Healthy or saturated fats such as coconut oil, avocado oil, olive oil, chia seeds, wild caught salmon

-Collagen, such as bone broth

- Fermented foods such as, Kefir, Sauerkraut, Kombucha, sourdough, yogurt

-Easily digestible foods such as chicken, turkey, fish, cooked fruits and vegetables, soups, smoothies, and purees

10

The Gut Microbiome

Your gut microbiome is an ecosystem living within your intestines. It's occupied by trillions of microorganisms that each play different roles within your body's function as a whole. There are thousands of species of bacteria, viruses, fungi, and parasites. These microorganisms have a symbiotic relationship with us as their occupants. We provide them with sustenance and a place for them to live and they provide important services for our bodies. You can think of it as a garden. Tended to, and needs fulfilled will yield a beautiful bounty. Tarnish its soil, neglect it and throw chemicals on it and it would upset the whole ecosystem.

A healthy microbiome aids our bodies in digestion. certain bacteria helps to break down our food we can't for ourselves, such as the lactose I mentioned before. This also explains why some are not intolerant to the lactose. Gut bacteria also helps metabolize bile in your intestines. You're liver sends bile to your small intestine to aid in digesting fats. Consequently bacteria and their enzymes help to break it down so that the bile acids can be reabsorbed and recycled by your liver. This process is known as enterohepatic circulation.

A thriving microbiome also plays a substantial role in our Immunity, nervous and endocrine systems.

So what can we do to help our own individual Gut ecosystems thrive? Here are a few great places to start.

1. Find a good quality probiotic and prebiotic
2. Increase your food diversity with a variety of plant rich and whole foods such as whole grains vegetables and fruits
3. Avoid the use of antibiotics as much as possible. A large percentage of antibiotics are prescribed unnecessarily. When doctors prescribe them they usually always say they'll be prescribing an antibiotic *just in case*. When in reality they have no idea if you have an infection because they didn't do the testing necessary to know if you have one. The whole point of an antibiotic is to kill everything. That's like dropping an atomic bomb right in the middle of that beautiful garden you and your body work so hard to help thrive. Don't mistake my opinion of antibiotics to be that they have no place. They definitely do and it can be a life saving drug when an infection is clearly present. All I'm saying is that taking them as a precautionary measure should be avoided at all costs.

11

Healing and Happiness Can Be Yours Too

I said a lot of things in these chapters, and I'm hoping most, if not all of it made sense to you and got your gears moving about all the possibilities that are yours to start on your journey to restore or improve your gut health. And in turn give your body healing in so many other areas as a result. So let's sum this up shall we? If I only had 1 minute to explain what hacks and first steps you should take to get started it would be this.

Figure out how to decrease inflammation in your gut starting with your diet, and lower your physical and emotional stress. Eliminate all processed foods, and Inflammatory oils and replace them with a nutrient dense and diverse diet of natures food. As well as making the difficult decisions in your life that could result in a lighter happier you. I'd then tell you to get a good probiotic and eat more fermented foods to aid in nurturing your gut microbiome. Getting a good quality digestive enzyme to give your body a boost in breaking down your food. Since in disrepair your gut is unable to perform that function optimally without a little bit of help.

These were all actions that I took vigorously in the beginning of my healing journey that have now become a seamless part of my everyday

23

life. Not just seeing, but feeling the progress my body has made not only makes my way of living crucial for me ,but it's become something I truly and enjoy and have a deep passion about now. My hope is that through my experiences you can find a more fast tracked trail to improving your gut and overall health.

I'm not going to lie. It was a solid year of following these very pieces of advice to a tee. And since it was a new way of living for me it wasn't always easy. But guess what, since healing my gut and sealing those perforations. My body functions as it was always intended to. Now, I eat my fair share of Texas Roadhouse rolls, and can enjoy a big Andy's concrete from time to time. I no longer limit myself much to what I can and can't eat. I have helped my body enough that it can now handle these things, and process them as god designed. My general rule of thumb is that I do really well at home. We don't buy anything that could cause harm to my family's guts and health in an environment we have full control over. But whenever I'm out, or on vacation I simply don't have to worry about it. I truly feel free. Whereas before I was confined to the rim of the small bowl that held my sad portion of rice. I haven't been bloated for over a year. My energy has increased, my thirst for life and happiness has never been more vibrant. I feel lighter. Metaphorically and physically. I now enjoy weight management and have not veered but 1-3 pounds through the year. I no longer feel nauseous or experience pain during digestion. All tell tale signs that my body is pleased with me. It's grateful for me ,and the decisions I've made to give us a better, healthier life. Let me emphasize. THIS CAN BE YOUR STORY TOO. Recognizing the need for better gut health is the first step in the right direction. Now put one foot in front of the other by following these natural, simple lifestyle changes. I promise by doing so and being consistent, you will start to see the effects in one way or another. Or better yet, complete healing, wholeness, and happiness within your body. Believe in yourself and the process. You've got this.

Hope, happiness, and health are ahead.

12

Resources

Schirm, A. (2023, March 27). *What is Metabolic Eating? Every Detail You Need*. The Living Well. https://thelivingwell.com/what-is-metabolic-eating-every-detail-you-need/

Professional, C. C. M. (n.d.). *Leaky Gut Syndrome*. Cleveland Clinic. https://my.clevelandclinic.org/health/diseases/22724-leaky-gut-syndrome

Rdn, D. L. M. (2024, January 6). *7 Sneaky signs you have leaky gut syndrome, according to a dietitian*. EatingWell. https://www.eatingwell.com/sneaky-signs-of-leaky-gut-syndrome-8421526

Schmanski, M. (2023, April 18). *The top foods to avoid for a healthy gut*. Gastroenterology Consultants of San Antonio. https://www.gastroconsa.com/the-top-foods-to-avoid-for-a-healthy-gut/

Campos, M., MD. (2023, September 12). *Leaky gut: What is it, and what does it mean for you?* Harvard Health. https://www.health.harvard.edu/blog/leaky-gut-what-is-it-and-what-does-it-mean-for-you-2017092212451

Chronic inflammation: Why its harmful and how to Prevent it. (2022, February 10). https://www.novanthealth.org/healthy-headlines/chronic-inflammation-why-its-harmful-and-how-to-prevent-it. https://www.novanthealth.org/healthy-headlines/chronic-inflammation-why-its-harmful-and-how-to-prevent-it

Mj, S. P. (2024, March 7). *Top 8 American foods banned in other countries.* Xtalks. https://xtalks.com/top-8-american-foods-banned-in-other-countries-3495/

Xenos, C. (2021, November 3). Common US foods that are banned in other countries. *Chicago Tribune.* https://www.chicagotribune.com/2021/11/03/common-us-foods-that-are-banned-in-other-countries/

NASD - Stress management for the health of it. (n.d.). https://nasdonline.org/1445/d001245/stress-management-for-the-health-of-it.html#:~:text=You%20can%20become%20negatively%20influenced,and%20disease%20is%20stress%2Drelated.

Professional, C. C. M. (n.d.-a). *Gut microbiome.* Cleveland Clinic. https://my.clevelandclinic.org/health/body/25201-gut-microbiome

www.ingramcontent.com/pod-product-compliance
Lightning Source LLC
Chambersburg PA
CBHW070755260726
48660CB00007B/3141

9 798884 556690